Alcohol Control

A Complete Guide For Overcoming Alcohol Addiction, Detoxifying the Body of Alcohol, and Discovering True Freedom in Life

Evelyn Cribster

ISBN: 978-1-63750-177-1

Table of Contents

Introduction

Detoxification is the first stage of drug abuse recovery. It entails a period after your last drink that you devote to ridding all the alcoholic beverages or toxins within you to be able to start treatment with a clean slate. When you stop drinking, it takes up to 10 days for the alcohol to altogether leave your system. It's a tricky time. Most people struggle in the early days. You get cravings, and your thinking becomes emotional. The principal goal of detoxification is to securely and comfortably begin an interval of abstinence at the beginning of the healing process.

Many people question whether drinking has become too big a part of their lives and worry that it may even be affecting their health. But they resist change because they fear losing the pleasure and stress relief associated with alcohol and assume giving it up will involve deprivation and misery.

Changing your habits can be hard without the right tools. This is especially true for alcohol because habits are, by definition, subconscious thought processes. Through her methodical research of the latest neuroscience and her own journey, this Author has cracked the code on habit change by addressing the specific ways habits form. This unique and unprecedented method has now helped thousands redefine their relationship to drinking painlessly and without misery.

This book walks you through the detox period painlessly and explains everything you need to achieve your sobriety short or long term goal.

Chapter 1

WHAT IS DETOXIFICATION?

Detoxification is the first stage of drug abuse recovery. It entails a period after your last drink that you devote to ridding all the alcoholic beverages or toxins within you to be able to start treatment with a clean slate. The principal goal of detoxification is to securely and comfortably begin an interval of abstinence at the beginning of the healing process. Research demonstrates the conclusion of medical alcoholic beverages detoxification, escalates the likelihood of successful treatment. Once the body is free from the short-term ramifications of alcoholic beverages, recovery will start.

Why is it essential to detox properly from alcoholic beverages?

Alcoholic beverages can be one of the most dangerous substances to withdraw. As cleansing progresses, withdrawal symptoms could become life-threatening, so healthcare monitoring is essential often for misuse and dependency. As the importance of actually ridding yourself of the consequences, alcohol is pressured in detoxification. It is important to judge for just about any of the psychological factors that often accompany severe alcohol dependence, such as depressed feeling, anxiety, and disposition swings, since research implies that such conditions complicate treatment and make successful treatment not as likely.

Some detoxification facilities, especially luxury programs that can offer one-on-one care, may evaluate patients for co-occurring psychiatric conditions during cleansing so that any mental medical issues can be appropriately managed.

Alcohol cleansing can be uncomfortable until withdrawal symptoms are in order. Withdrawal could possibly be the most difficult area of the treatment process. Patients who have involved in heavy, long term drinking are suffering from physical reliance on alcoholic beverages and rely on it to activate the body's regulatory functions.

Alcohol Withdrawal: Physical Symptoms

Patience experience alcoholic beverages withdrawal differently. However, most people will experience at least a few of the following severe alcohol withdrawal symptoms:

- Racing pulse

- Increased blood circulation pressure

- Fever

- Sweating

- Headache

- Mood swings

- Anxiety

- Confusion

- Agitation

- Seizures

Seizures will be the most dangerous of acute alcoholic beverages withdrawal symptoms. They happen because the human brain and the cellular material within it have transformed as they have become familiar with the persistent existence of alcoholic beverages and its sedating effects on your system.

When alcohol is abruptly taken off your system, your body cannot access chemicals that assist your central nervous system calm itself after being excited. The human brain challenges to change to the rebounding degree of activation. Sometimes the mind can't match all of this new excitatory neuronal activity, which can lead to a seizure.

The chance of experiencing an alcohol-related seizure peak at 24-48 hours following the last drink remains high. In some instances, several times from then on.

Therefore, it is essential to your treatment course that you start with detox and also have all the alcohol taken off the body first. For some, starting treatment for alcoholic beverages abuse after properly completing cleansing is the ultimate way to get yourself to accomplish sobriety. That way, the most literally uncomfortable part has ended, and you may focus your time and efforts on recovery.

What to Expect

The severity of the person's withdrawal during detox is closely related to how severe and long-standing he has been addicted. It's important to bear in mind that your connection with detoxification may vary from what you read here or what you might have observed in other people. Just how your cleansing advances will be affected by many factors, so it's difficult to determine with precision what course your detoxification may take.

However, you'll be able to get an over-all timeframe for the detox process, filled with the progression of symptoms.

The First Hours of Alcoholic Beverages Detox

Cravings are a few of the first symptoms of alcoholic beverages withdrawal, and a definitive indication that your body is starting the cleansing process.

- Cravings may appear within hours of going for the last drink and continue much into the detoxification process.

The first hours of cleansing could also involve symptoms such as:

- Nausea and vomiting.

- Anxiety, restlessness, depressive disorder, or irritability.

- Spikes in heart rate and blood circulation pressure.

- Nightmares and insomnia.

- Tremors (quite common for all those levels of alcoholic beverages addiction).

For patients with an increase of extensive physical reliance on alcoholic beverages, symptoms may persist and get progressively worse throughout the withdrawal process.

The First Two Times of Alcoholic Beverages Detox

Following the initial hours of untreated alcohol withdrawal, more acute severe symptoms are possible.

As well as the symptoms explained above, new symptoms at this time range from hallucinations and seizures.

The symptoms that develop within the first two times of detox may become life-threatening if the mind struggles to compensate for having less chemical indicators to re-enter the resting normal physical condition after anxiety or enjoyment and can lose its control over heart rate, blood circulation pressure, and nervous system activity.

- Hallucinations are possible in this stage of detoxification.

- Seizures are possible as well, mostly in the first 12 to 48 hours following the last drink, but can continue for times following the process starts.

- Rapid heart rate and high blood circulation

pressure continue if no intervention occurs.

- Chest pain may arise, which might indicate insufficient blood circulation to the center (thanks to increased blood circulation pressure and also to the heart's higher energy importance).

- Delirium tremens: a severe, dangerous aftereffect of acute alcoholic beverages withdrawal (see below for symptoms).

- For most, the cleansing process will not end at 48 hours.

- Severe or long-standing instances of alcoholic beverages addiction may necessitate particularly close monitoring for times, following the decision to detoxify has begun.

All of those other Alcohol Detox Process

Detoxification can continue for most days following the preliminary withdrawal symptoms develop, which urges, restlessness, and anxiety intensify with long exercises of untreated alcoholic beverages withdrawal. If present, rather than managed carefully, seizure activity may upsurge in severity and rate of recurrence.

Following the first 48 hours of detox, seizure risk will start to reduce often. However, continuing medical observation may be important as the chance of extreme misunderstandings and cardiovascular occasions such as coronary attack and heart stroke remain elevated.

If an individual experiences these results, symptoms usually occur within 48 to 96 hours following the last drink. Sometimes, they have a postponed starting point, starting between 7 and 10 times following the last drink.

Delirium tremens (DT) medical indications include:

- Body tremors.

- Agitation or irritability.

- Fever and perspiration.

- Extreme confusion or disorientation.

- Quick mood changes.

- Hallucinations.

- Seizures.

Since DT is a dangerous condition with a higher death rate, it is almost always managed within an inpatient medical hospital's intensive treatment device. Mortality rates in unmanaged situations of delirium tremens are 10-

15%. Sedating medications, diligent guidance, and supportive care and attention will make a difference until the health threats subside.

Risk Factors for Delirium Tremens

A man experiencing symptoms in Delirium tremens won't develop Atlanta divorce attorneys recovering alcohol consumer, but since it is so dangerous, you ought to have your physician or other addiction treatment professional, evaluate your risk to be able to best-plan potential problems. The rapidity of onset and intensity of DT symptoms depends on how much and exactly how ordinarily a person drink.

Risk factors for developing DT during alcoholic beverages withdrawal include:

- The cessation of taking in after a period of taking in heavily.

- Not wanting to eat enough food throughout an amount of chronic or heavy taking in.

- Head injury, infection, or illness in a person with a brief history of heavy taking in.

- History of alcoholic beverages withdrawal experiences.

- Drinking a lot or often to get more than a decade.

Alcohol cleansing and withdrawal can be physically and psychologically taxing health problems, cravings, and feeling swings are normal. It appears like frightening information, but it's important to be appropriately familiarized with the detoxification process, particularly when you have a severe dependency.

Can I Get it Done at Home?

Even if you'd choose to cleanse from alcohol at home, finding professional supervision is really important. Mild to moderate withdrawal symptoms can be handled on either an inpatient or outpatient basis, as research shows little difference in results between these configurations. When there is a risk for severe symptoms, alcoholic beverages withdrawal must be maintained in a severe medical establishing. Alcohol detoxification and withdrawal bring the chance of extreme health consequences, including hallucinations, seizures, and loss of life. Finding an effective cleansing program, whether it is conducted with an inpatient or outpatient basis-is paramount to your recovery security.

You will find outpatient recovery programs that enable you to sort out recovery from your home. Nevertheless, you should seek advice from your doctor before investing in outpatient detox, as it might not be the most likely option if you are in risk for physical withdrawal symptoms or you have other circumstances that could jeopardize your recovery efforts.

Relatively mild symptoms of withdrawal may be managed if aware of appropriate medications and frequent check-ins with a supervising physician. However, it is difficult to forecast withdrawal advancements, and further, difficult to control for all your factors at home. For these and other reasons, going through detoxification at a service and then working through the others of treatment from your home is a superb option for most in early recovery.

Alcohol Detox Treatment

Lots of the symptoms of acute alcoholic beverages withdrawal will have largely faded after five times of detox, while some may persist for weeks or longer. Any serious symptoms still present at this time will be clinically handled at the cleansing center.

Clinically assisted detoxification involves professional health monitoring through the detox phase to make sure your safety throughout the risky alcohol withdrawal effects. Traditional treatment will provide you with supportive therapy that will assist prepare you for time for everyday living and demonstrate how to manage drinking temptations effectively.

Luxury treatment also provides quality drug abuse

treatment, but these facilities additionally place concentrate on personal privacy and comfort. In an extravagance or professional program. You'll find many amenities i.e. private rooms, access to the internet, leisure entertainment, and more one-on-one treatment.

Because alcoholic beverages detoxification, withdrawal, and recovery can at first be this uncomfortable process, luxury configurations are perfect for those in recovery from alcoholic beverages addiction. Many choose to go through treatment in the best luxury home rehabilitation programs in the united states, where they'll also receive mental counseling and support from others in recovery.

Traditional treatment programs use similar therapeutic methods and can just be as beneficial as luxury rehabs are to the people in recovery. The number of amenities may be less than those at the blissful luxury centers. However, the treatment services are generally offered at a lesser cost. Whatever your decision, ensure that you put your wellbeing first; both physical and mental, throughout the procedure.

Chapter 2

How to Detox from Alcohol from Home

If you have browsed the cautionary caution in the preceding section but still wish to go after self-detox from alcoholic beverages, here are lots of preliminary steps that are important to undertake to ensure the procedure is safe, and also to increase its likelihood of success:

- Remove ALL alcohol consumption from your home; this is an essential step.

- Clear the routine, create enough time necessary for complete detoxing, could take several weeks. Make sure nothing at all stands in ways.

- Get active support, finances for it with family or

friends who'll make sure a detoxing person is Okay, and who'll be there if the average person needs anything.

- Concentrate on hydration, make sure a detoxing person drinks enough liquid because this will rehydrate your body and be rid of toxins.

- Take vitamins, B-complex, Niacin, vitamin C, magnesium, and zinc. Test to see which work best.

Main Types of Self-Detox from Alcohol

- *Cold Turkey*: fast, abrupt, more painful way to avoid alcohol consumption

- *Tapering Off*: steadily preventing, using less and less alcohol

Alcohol detoxification can be carried out at home, but not under some circumstances.

Alcohol cleansing at home is usually safe for the binge-drinker who only celebrate on weekends because their bodies have not developed the full-blown addiction. These drinkers could become significantly uncomfortable while trying self-detox from alcoholic beverages, but probably this discomfort won't transfer to the life-threatening category.

This is also true of the "Tapering Off" method of self-detox. It could be done securely When there is another person presently monitoring the number of alcoholic beverages consumed, and If the individual is permitted to drink only a drink with a lesser alcoholic beverages content, like ale, and If this usage is doled out by the supervisor only. If the alcohol-dependent person is left to monitor himself or herself, generally, the person will increase usage to steer clear of the pain of withdrawal.

The Cool Turkey Approach

Lady in despair addresses her face with hands sitting down on the couch "Cool Turkey" implies sudden secession of alcoholic beverages consumption. This technique can succeed for some since it quickens the road to recovery. It is much harder than the next "Tapering Off" method, but they have shown to be a good choice for some.

It's important to comprehend, however, that withdrawal symptoms can be quite severe. The body of the alcoholic is familiar with huge amounts of alcoholic beverages, which explains why abrupt discontinuation of intake can become a surprise to your body. The Cool Turkey method can cause the next withdrawal symptoms:

- Nausea

- Headaches

- Insomnia

- Sweating

- Heartrate increase

- Hallucinations (audio-visual-tactile)

- Fever

- Seizures.

The Tapering Off Approach

Tapering off is a way of alcoholic beverages detoxification that includes slow reduction of one's amount of daily alcoholic beverages intake. It is a less severe strategy in regards to negative effects such as belly aches and pains, nausea, and other unpleasant symptoms. Many people choose beverage as a tapering off tool, so if one is an ale lover, this may work in their favor. If indeed they opt because of this cleansing method, be sure to limit a regular alcohol intake regularly rather than fluctuate backward and forwards.

Overall, alcoholic beverages home detoxification is neither the very best nor the safest approach to quitting alcoholic beverages addiction; however, in some instances, it can be an inexpensive and effective one.

Having someone around to ensure a detoxing is specific and steady, and always a good notion, so if one chooses to endure self-detox from alcoholic beverages, they ought to remind their finest friend, family, or perhaps a doctor to be sure of them regularly, in the event. That is essential if a person desires to apply safe alcohol detoxification at home.

Risks of Alcoholic Beverages Detox at Home

The potential risks of alcohol detoxification at home far outweigh the huge benefits for several reasons. First, detoxing at home is hardly ever successful. A lot of people quit the procedure and resume consuming within the first day, just from the issue of controlling the symptoms. An area of concern would be that the alcoholic doesn't have the support at home that he/she could have at the cure center. There's an importance for guidance, friends, helpful mentors, and group support that is seldom present in the house situation, and definitely not present in 24 hours per day, 7 days weekly. The drinker could use important medical assistance because of the life-threatening physical and emotional symptoms that can occur during detox.

Side Effects of Detoxing from Alcoholic beverages at Home

Just like a reminder why the response to the question "How to safely detox from alcohol at home" it is important to know that "One can't always make sure it'll be safe," Common side ramifications of self-detox include:

- Pacing, restlessness, and irritability.

- Agitation

- High blood circulation pressure

- Muscle cramps, body pain, and tremors

- Increased heart rate

- Diarrhea and other intestinal crises

- Hypoglycemia or low bloodstream sugar level

- Headaches, dizziness, and confusion

- Hot and cold flashes changes of body's temperature.

Physical Symptoms

Oftentimes, it's the serious and disabling physical symptoms of detox that change the drinker's brain about, continuing with the procedure. These symptoms tend to be severe and should preferably be supervised by medical personnel. Some physical problems include:

- The necessity to maneuver around, restlessness and irritability

- Feeling as though your skin is crawling and being agitated

- Blood circulation pressure can increase to high levels

- Pains and shakes, and feeling as though "every muscle hurts" as alcoholic beverages are flushed from the system

- Pulse rate raises with the strain of the withdrawal

- The digestive tract moves into crisis; diarrhea is

common

- The blood sugars drop because alcohol is a kind of sugar in the torso

- The average person may have symptoms of hypoglycemia

- Headaches, dizziness, and confusion

- Tiredness, heat changes in the torso, hot and cool flashes

- Shaking and cramping muscles.

Psychological Symptoms

There may be serious psychological symptoms as well, including:

- Generalized anxiety sense just like a hammer is

dangling over the top, and bad things tend to happen

- Hallucinations

- Intense urges to get relief

- Feeling like your body is arriving apart.

- Feeling swings - from anxiety, to hopelessness, to suicidal

- Paranoia often accompanies the hallucinations and can escalate into defensive actions.

Delirium Tremens

Delirium Tremens (the DTs) will be the most dangerous withdrawal sign for alcoholics, with the probability of them occurring to at least 1 in 10 individuals in withdrawal. The death count from serious situations of DTs is often as high as 35%.

The symptoms of delirium tremens may appear within 72 hours of alcohol withdrawal and can appear without warning. DTs can occur anytime during the withdrawal period but will present through the first ten times.

Indicators of delirium tremens during self-detox include:

- Grand mal seizures, seen as a loss of awareness and violent muscle contractions

- Jeopardized heart functions including high blood circulation pressure, suppressed deep breathing, and low oxygen levels

- Hallucinations

- Paranoia

- Confusion

- Anxiety and agitation

DTs medical treatment and monitoring is important because they have many dangerous characteristics, such as:

- Grand mal seizures, where an individual can thrash about, swallow their tongue or bite it off, lose awareness, or become physically hyper-strong.

- Heart functions can be compromised as pulse rate and blood circulation pressure rises, and deep breathing may be suppressed, which in turn causes the oxygen source to the cardiovascular to diminish. The probability of heart stroke or coronary attack is increased.

- The alcoholic experiencing DTs may have hallucinations such as bugs crawling on the skin or spiders in the area. They could claw at their encounters and rip at their pores and skin. The average person can also do long term harm to their eye, thinking that their eye has become broken because of the hallucinations.

- The alcoholic may become paranoid and attack someone because they believe they may be being hunted or threatened.

- The alcoholic will be confused by the sugar withdrawal, which can lead to impaired judgment in critical situations.

- The average person may be anxious and agitated, unable to cope with social situations.

Reasons people take the risk of continuing to drink

The number one reason that people with alcohol abuse problems continue to drink is that they believe they "have it under control." This is a dangerous thought because these individuals are likely to die from alcohol poisoning, like Amy Winehouse. The following are the most cited reasons why someone continues with their addictive behavior:

- **Denial:** They deny the problem, ignore their behavior, and withdraw from criticism and those that confront them with their addiction issues.

- **Lack of control at a treatment center:** They

want to control the issue themselves as they have already lost control of their bodies and relationships.

- **Fear of change in their lives:** They fear the pain and discomfort of withdrawal and the process of rehabilitation. Any type of change moves them out of their "comfort zone."

- **Fear of life:** The individual knows that they don't have the coping skills to have a normal life, so they choose a dysfunctional pattern. It may be bad, but it is better than appearing inadequate.

- **Self-defeating attitude:** Many people with alcohol dependency believes there isn't help and hope. These people need important mental health treatment and counselling for depression, simultaneous with addiction rehab

- **Stigma:** Many people fear "what other people will think" if they go to rehab for help. They don't realize that these "other people" they're worried about already notice the addiction problem.

- **The desire to die:** The addicted individual has lost the desire to live and is using alcohol to commit a form of "slow suicide." This type of person will drink until they die unless they receive an unwanted intervention.

- **Cost:** Many alcoholics will say that the cost is too prohibitive for them to seek professional help through a rehab center, but this is erroneous. Insurance will cover 30 days of rehab, Medicare will cover 30 days, and if someone has no insurance at all, a judge can order rehab at no cost to the individual seeking help.

Chapter 3

9 Ways of Cleansing After a Long Night

1. Sleep in.

A hangover is actually the biological taxes you purchase after partying. There's no real remedy, but sleeping through the most severe of it is an excellent spot to start. Plus, though alcoholic beverages make you drift off quickly, it offers you crap rest.

2. Drink a lot of water.

It's likely that, if you went big on cocktails yesterday evening, you're probably incredibly dehydrated right now, which will make you feel drained and having a headache. Blame it on the alcohol because it's a diuretic.

3. Intensify the rehydration with electrolytes.

Gatorade, coconut drinking water, and Pedialyte (the children's drink and hardcore partier's key tool) contain electrolytes, including sodium and potassium, that help the body hold onto water.

4. Eat eggs for breakfast

Both alcoholic beverages and mixers are saturated in glucose; a hangover is within large part an enormous sugars crash. Your blood glucose can decrease to virtually zero. So it's important to get some good food back into one's body. Eggs contain cysteine, an amino acid that counteracts a harmful byproduct of alcoholic beverages' metabolism. Can't take it in? Start with something like crackers, grain, or broth.

5. Sip some ginger tea.

It can help quell nausea and could also reduce any lingering dizziness. Plus, it's just very soothing. And drink water. You will have to prioritize taking enough water.

6. Add honey

Fructose has been proven (anecdotally and in a few research) to accelerate alcoholic beverages metabolism in the torso. Honey provides you a good fructose value for your money. (So eat a few of that, too.)

7. Get a walk and get some good fresh air.

The claims that o_2 relieves hangover symptoms are sketchy at best (remember air pubs?), though many people swear the bond is real. Walk in the new air and get the breathing going just a little. More o_2 moving through your veins can only just help your liver organ with the monumental job of filtering the harmful toxins from alcoholic beverages out of your bloodstream. Plus, it'll get you out of your stuffy apartment and it'll feel great to be up and about.

8. Ramp it up to jog or engage other forms of exercise.

"Working out produces endorphins (disposition enhancers), which can only help you feel better faster," Beth Recanati, M.D., a women's health and fitness specialist, tells Personal. Try out this twisty yoga exercise routine for your day after a particular large date to wring yourself out, just like a dishtowel.

9. When your belly is designed for it, eat meats, coffee beans, and lentils.

Chapter 4

Alcohol Detoxification: 10 Natural Methods to be Healthier after Boozing'

Stay on the Wagon; Destination: Balance

America and arguably a large area of the world - is soaked in booze, making an alcohol cleansing challenging for individuals who dread they've crossed the collection between party and problem.

Based on the Countrywide Council on Alcoholism and Medicine Dependence (NCADD), alcoholic beverages are the most used addictive material in America: 17.6 million people, or one Atlanta divorce attorney (12 adults), is suffering from alcoholic beverages mistreatment or dependence. In the meantime, several million take part in dangerous, binge consuming patterns.

Just about any interpersonal gathering revolves around booze, from frat celebrations to one-night time stands, making alcoholic beverages difficult to withstand even when you understand that it's filled up with sugar and will be offering no real benefits. Reducing or kicking your alcoholic beverages habit completely may be important in repairing balance to your wellbeing and adding years to your daily life. Alcohol detox will help you do this.

Dangers of Moderates Alcohol Consumption

Alcoholic beverages can directly harm the liver organ, intestines, digestive tract, stomach, and esophagus while increasing the probability of creating a laundry set of cancers, partly because of its higher sugar content. Dr. Robert Lustig proved in a 2015 study that sugar is "toxic regardless of its calories and regardless of its weight."

When you consume alcohol, the body reacts to it as a toxin and throws its energy into eliminating it. This means that other processes are disrupted, including glucose production, especially in the liver and the hormones to regulate it. Interfering with the liver's production of glucose can cause problems such as hypoglycemia. Alcohol also includes ethanol, a substance that can transform the mitochondrial structure, which plays a vital role in alcohol metabolism. Additionally, it may affect the function of several organs, like the liver and the heart.

You don't have to drink a lot of alcohol for this to have unwanted effects. Even moderate alcohol consumption can boost the risk of breast cancer, promote mental decline, and impact pregnancy. For example, premenopausal women who consume 10 ounces (a little glass) of wine, an 8-ounce beer, or an ounce of hard liquor each day have a 5 percent greater potential for getting breast cancer. That number jumps to 9 percent for post-menopausal women, according to a written report from the American Institute for Cancer Research and the World Cancer Research Fund. So when you take these into account, roughly 12 percent of ladies in America and the UK will have breast cancer sooner or later in their lifetimes, that's a substantial upsurge in risk.

Furthermore, experts from the University of Oxford and London discovered that there's a correlation between moderate drinking and mental decline. Results of their 30-year study showed that individuals who consumed high degrees of alcohol were at an elevated risk for

Hippocampal atrophy, a kind of brain damage often associated with memory-loss conditions like Alzheimer's and dementia, which moderates that drinkers are 3times more likely to have Hippocampal atrophy than people who didn't drink.

Another new research showed that taking in smaller amounts of alcohol when pregnant could change a child's features. Experts found that alcoholic beverages affected face shape, specifically around the nose, eyes, and lips, when consumed throughout the pregnancy and in the first trimester.

Why an Alcoholic Beverages Detox?

Despite its dangers, moderate and heavy alcohol consumption is sticking around. In 2015, Millennial drank more than 42 percent of most wine in America, according to a report from your wine Market Council. Even the rise in popularity and legalization of recreational marijuana in America hasn't negatively impacted alcohol consumption and sales. Colorado tax records show that both developed a pseudo symbiotic relationship, steadily increasing side-by-side.

In case your "one drink" often becomes three or four, you might be damaging your pancreas, tampering with your body's sugar levels, reducing communication in the middle of your brain as well as your body, developing an emotional or physical dependency, putting yourself at risk of developing liver disease, and more. You might be putting some nasty toxins within you. For instance, a report discovered that 14 popular German beers are filled with glyphosate, the active component in Monsanto's weed-killer Roundup, and it's likely within other beers which have not been investigated.

Natural Alcohol Cleansing Methods

So, what can we do to fight the consequences of constant alcohol consumption? Everything starts with alcohol detox. This is done in a hospital, but you're guaranteed to be pumped with medications that are cross-tolerant with alcohol and include their group of risks such as benzodiazepines (anti-anxiety medications) and anticonvulsants. Thankfully, nature has come through for all of us once again by giving incredible herbs, plants, vitamins, and minerals like passionflower, milk thistle, vitamin B, and activated charcoal that facilitate an all-natural alcohol detox process. The next methods don't reverse the damage of ongoing alcoholism; however, they can kick start your wellbeing journey, whether you want to:

- Overcome a hangover

- Scale back on occasional drinking

- Stop binge drinking

- Stop consuming completely

For those who drink occasionally or want to eliminate a hangover, focus on numbers two, three, five, and ten below. For all those targeting alcohol withdrawal symptoms from binge drinking, focus on numbers one, eight, and six. If you're trying to give up completely, pay special focus on numbers four, five, seven, and nine. Never make an effort to detox without medical supervision. A specialist can help you select what's best for the body, and which mixture of alcohol detox methods are best for you.

Here are ten (10) natural alcohol detoxification methods:

1. Drink Passion Blossom Tea

Many people experience insomnia and anxiety during an alcohol detox since when your body undergoes a withdrawal of alcohol, a substance used to function with, and it is often used to self-medicate anxiety, the human brain starts new chemicals and neurotransmitters that put extra stress on your brain function. Ultimately, this leads to anxiety, which can cause restlessness and disrupted sleep patterns.

Drinking flower tea or passionflower extract can improve the quality of sleep and anxiety levels. Research implies that passionflower is a highly effective treatment for insomnia, so when coupled with herbs like valerian, hops, and lemon balm is even more efficient. Top-quality products such as these are from Native Remedies Pure Calm (with passionflower, lemon balm and lavender (with passionflower, kava, and St. John's Wort) as well as for sound sleep:

Another study discovered that enthusiasm blossom helped alleviate anxiety associated with alcoholic beverages withdrawals. When analysts offered alcohol-addicted mice experiencing withdrawals interest flower extract, the mice's withdrawal anxiety was reduced by 90 percent in comparison to mice that didn't have the extract.

2. Essential Oils

The first stages of your cleansing process will probably include fighting withdrawal. Janice Rosenthal, the owner of the Garden of Essences and aromatherapy expert, suggests organic essential oils to soothe your experience. She recommends mixing 15 drops of body butter and putting it on to your upper abdomen, sides, and back. That is a powerful do-it-yourself solution, which works rapidly to detoxify the liver, as the fundamental oils permeate your skin and reach the liver's bloodstream directly within around 30 minutes," Rosenthal explains.

3. B-complex vitamins

Alcohol consumption can cause the body to burn off through B vitamins quicker than normal. Replenishing the body with B-complex nutritional vitamins like B-1, B-3, and B-5 reduces alcohol withdrawal symptoms and supports the detoxification process. Research demonstrates vitamin B-1, a vitamin that alcoholics are generally deficient in.

It can lessen fatigue and increase effective brain functioning, while vitamin B-5 helps eliminate alcohol within you and supports adrenal function. According to Dr. Alex Roher, M.D., vitamin B-3 can also relieve the symptoms of alcohol withdrawal like cravings and insomnia. "Niacin (vitamin B-3) can be especially effective in larger recommended doses," Roher says.

4. Activated Charcoal

Turned on charcoal is a robust vitamin that works to fully capture chemicals and toxins in the torso, rendering it a great detoxifier. Qualified Nutritional Specialist, Renee Belz, highly recommends activated charcoal for detoxing from alcohol. "My absolute No.1 (alcohol detox vitamin) is charcoal. It binds toxins in the GI tract (especially alcohol)," she says.

Belz claims that activated charcoal is effective before and after consuming alcohol. However, studies also show that it may significantly reduce blood alcohol concentrations when taken at precisely the same time as alcohol. Belz says that typical protocol demands 1,000 to 2,000 mg of activated charcoal.

5. Add Milk Thistle

Milk thistle established the fact for being an all-natural liver organ detoxifier and is often recommended as an all-natural remedy for alcoholic beverages detoxification. Although, research implies that milk thistle may regenerate damaged liver tissue, remove toxins in the torso, and block the absorption of alcohol in the liver. Belz explains that milk thistle dosage may differ based on body weight, but the typical protocol is 50 mg of the potent liver detoxifier. You can consume the milk thistle plant's leaves and seeds in powder, pill, tea, tincture, or extract form. Liver tonics with milk thistle as a primary ingredient, provide comprehensive liver detoxification.

6. Put in a Dash Of Cayenne

Adding cayenne pepper to your meal or going for a single drop dose may help alleviate alcohol withdrawal symptoms. Dr. Samuel Malloy, director at DrFelix and expert in holistic medicine, recommends cayenne pepper for common symptoms. "Cayenne pepper may boost your appetite, and it comes with unpleasant withdrawal symptoms like nausea," says Malloy.

"Additionally, it may decrease the pain of any tummy problems due to drinking excessive levels of alcohol, because it's saturated in anti-inflammatory substances." Cayenne pepper can also reduce inflammation of the stomach lining that's caused by excessive alcohol consumption. Check it out in its natural, powdered, cream, or capsule form to reap the advantages of its detoxifying properties!

7. Benefits from Kudzu

Kudzu main is a normal Chinese herb that is traditionally found in Japan and Southeast Asia to reduce various side ramifications of excessive alcohol consumption (hangovers, thirst, etc.). However, recent research demonstrates kudzu root vitamins, which are filled with potent antioxidants known as phytochemicals, which can curb alcohol cravings. A placebo-controlled double-blind human study discovered that participants who received kudzu root drank a significantly fewer quantity of beers than those who received the placebo.

Its antioxidant properties can also lessen overall liver harm and regenerate damaged liver organ. One study demonstrated that kudzu root extract stimulated liver regeneration and made the liver more resistant in adult male rats subjected to a chemical that triggers liver toxicity (carbon tetrachloride). If you don't want to consider it as a vitamin, check it out as a powder. Sneak it into the next sauce or soup!

8. Try Robuvit - French Oak Wooden Extract

Natural health physician and author Dr. Fred Pescatore, suggests a French oak wood extract, as an all-natural way to detox from alcohol. Research implies that Robuvit helps support the liver's natural detox function by eliminating toxins faster. Pescatore says that "whenever we consume alcohol, the short-term overload may exceed the liver's capacity to process and filter, which can result in the typical "hangover" effects most are acquainted with."

A new study demonstrates Robuvit® helps to protect the liver from alcohol-related damage and "to significantly improve symptoms of short-term hepatic damage including fatigue, nausea, and mild liver enlargement," Pescatore says. "It's safe, easy, and effective."

9. Angelica Extract

Angelica extract is a solid anti-inflammatory plant that can help reduce alcohol cravings and relieve withdrawal symptoms like headaches and bloating. It's also an antispasmodic agent, which smooth muscle spasms (particularly in the gastrointestinal tract), assisting the liver and spleen during long-term alcohol users' recovery processes. 3 to 5 drops in one glass of water usually does the secret. Be cautious with that one. Angelica extract will make you sick or nauseous if you go back to drinking.

10. Agua

It's vitally important to remain hydrated during any detox. Water really helps to flush out the toxins in one's body, replenish your body's water levels, and lessen the intensity of symptoms like withdrawal-related headaches.

Try mixing in a few lemon juices to increase your alcohol detox. Lemon water offers a healthy way to obtain vitamin C, helps restore your pH balance, and more. You might try coconut water. It adds alkalinity to the body, and it's abundant with potassium and other electrolytes and nutrients that can soothe an upset stomach or nausea.

Chapter 5

Natural Treatments for Alcoholism Addiction Treatment

Alcoholism Treatment and recovery are complicated procedures that require a lot of constant support. While it isn't recommended to rely exclusively on option therapies or remedies for the support, specific natural approaches can help improve your well-being while undergoing alcoholism treatment.

When Is Alcoholism Treatment Necessary?

Alcoholism, the popular term for alcoholic beverages dependence, is seen as several features, including craving, lack of control, physical dependence (typically triggering symptoms like nausea and sweating upon withdrawal), and tolerance.

However, because alcoholism can result in lots of friendly and emotional problems as well as serious health problems, it's essential to seek treatment if you have any observable symptoms of alcoholism (like a compulsion to drink or a failure to limit the quantity of alcohol you consume).

Natural Support

Certain natural substances and mind-body therapies show promise as a way of supporting your wellbeing while undergoing alcoholism treatment. If you are taking into consideration the use of these approaches, ensure that you discuss its potential benefits and dangers with the health-care experts involved with your alcoholism treatment.

Acupuncture for Alcoholic beverages Addiction

Acupuncture (an importance-based therapy long found in traditional Chinese language medication) is often recommended in reducing alcohol desires, relieve withdrawal symptoms, and simplify the panic and significant depression frequently experienced by alcoholics.

Indeed, a 2002 study of 34 alcoholics discovered that fourteen days of acupuncture treatments (coupled with carbamazepine; a drug sometimes found in managing alcohol withdrawal) helped reduce the participants' withdrawal symptoms. However, a systematic review published in '09 2009 figured there certainly insufficient evidence to aid acupuncture's effectiveness in alcoholism treatment.

Milk Thistle for Alcoholism

Milk thistle (Silybum marianum), a natural herb abundant with the antioxidant silymarin, is often touted as a way of restoring liver organ health and avoiding alcohol-induced liver organ damage. While research shows that milk thistle may offer some advantage to those seeking to treat alcohol-related liver organ disease, more studies had importance to attract any definitive conclusions about the herb's effectiveness in improving liver health.

Kudzu for Alcoholic beverages Dependence

In a 2003 research on lab rats, scientists found out that feeding the animals extract of kudzu (Pueraria lobata) helped curb their alcohol dependence. Also, little study released in 2005 demonstrated that taking kudzu vitamins helped reduce alcoholic beverages intake in humans.

The Importance of Alcoholism Treatment

With no help of alcoholism treatment, you might increase your threat of experiencing certain problems related to excessive drinking, including:

- Alcoholic hepatitis (inflammation of the liver organ)

- Cirrhosis (scarring of the liver organ)

- Gastritis (swelling of the liner of the belly)

- Pancreatitis

- High blood circulation pressure

- Bone loss

Furthermore, alcoholism has been associated with an elevated incidence of several cancers, including:

- Colon cancer

- Breast cancer

- Malignancy of the mouth area, neck, esophagus, larynx, and liver

Options for Alcoholism Treatment

Given the significant health threats associated with alcoholism, it is critical to seek alcoholism treatment only from professional healthcare with professional facilities.

Standard alcoholism treatment plans may start with detoxification, and perhaps involve home and outpatient programs that use several social supports.

C h a p t e r 6

The Very Best Diet For Alcohol Detox

Eating could be the very last thing you'll want to take into account as it pertains to alcoholic beverages detoxification. But since alcoholic beverages have a primary link with your body's capability to process and metabolize precise nutrition, you must start to feed the body with the food it needs to heal properly.

Through the initial phases of your cleansing, it might be difficult to consume any food whatsoever, but as your symptoms improve, it's essential to consume a well-balanced diet that will assist in bringing the body back to functional harmony. Below covers what types of foods, vitamins, and minerals you'll want relating to your diet plan after and during an alcohol cleansing.

1. Concentrate on Hydration

Through the initial levels of your alcohol cleanse, remaining hydrated is incredibly essential. The start phases of your alcoholic beverages drawback will generally induce a few of the following symptoms:

- Fatigue

- Anxiety

- Nausea/vomiting

- Lack of appetite

- Depression

- And more

Many of these symptoms will be worsened if you're also

dehydrated. Since alcoholic beverages dehydrate your body, you'll have to work doubly hard to make sure you give yourself a reliable supply of drinking water. Even though you are not thirsty, make an effort to drink water to help flush the body of toxins.

2. Eat Soups And Fluids During The Preliminary Detox

When you initially start your alcohol detoxification, which often lasts ranging from 24 and 72 hours, it could be challenging to keep food down. Don't pressure you to eat dense meals, even if they're healthy ultimately. Instead, concentrate on eating soups and other fluids to give the body some degree of sustenance.

If you're preparing the soups yourself, make sure they

contain a lot of vegetables, and even low-fat sources of proteins, such as coffee beans, poultry, or seafood. You can even drink teas and fruits and veggie juices to keep to give the body nutritional support.

3. Include Vitamin and Nutrient Support

A lot of people who are alcoholics commonly have some vitamin and nutrient deficiencies. Alcoholic beverages inhibit the body from effectively absorbing nutrition, including B nutritional vitamins. B nutritional vitamins are necessary for transforming food into functional energy. Common cleansing foods that contain B dietary vitamins include eggs, nut products, leafy greens, dairy, coffee beans, and fortified whole grains.

Other fat-soluble vitamins that you may be lacking

include:

- Vitamin A (within fish, carrots, dairy)

- Vitamin D (within the fortified dairy and fatty seafood)

- Vitamin E(within almonds, nut products, and natural vegetable oils)

- Vitamin K (within essential olive oil, and leafy greens)

It's essential to add an alcoholic beverage nutrient program throughout your detox to be able to help the body heal and recover quicker.

4. Implement A Well Balanced Diet

Since alcoholic beverages are heavy on sugars, it's

common for individuals detoxing from alcoholic beverages to crave sugary snack foods and sweets. Make an effort to reduce your usage of low-quality foods and only well-balanced meals that support you on your street to recovery. Even though you were a comparatively healthy eater when you were taking in, alcoholic beverages still impair your body's capability to make use of and break down essential nutrients.

A well-balanced diet includes a lot of healthy fruits & vegetables, lean resources of proteins like poultry and fish, whole grains, nuts, coffee beans, and low-fat dairy products. It's also important to add healthy natural oils such as essential olive oil and essential coconut oil.

If you're choosing a cure program to aid in your alcohol detox and recovery, it's essential that you choose a plan that includes dietary assistance and behavioral change within the program. This will increase your recovery and ease your changeover to a recently sober life.

5 Types Of Food To Consume When Detoxing From Alcohol

Withdrawal from alcoholic beverages is different for everybody and can last from a couple of days to a whole week. However, the cleansing stage (whenever a person is ridding oneself completely of alcoholic beverages) can last well following the end of the withdrawals, carrying on for a couple of weeks. Much like most situations in life, the body will react accordingly predicated on what you placed into it in this stage.

When detoxing, you'll be told that first and most

important is drinking water. Hydration is necessary generally, and particularly when withdrawing from alcoholic beverages as your body is modifying to less liquid intake than typical. But certain food organizations likewise have benefits as it pertains to the pain of withdrawals and detoxing. The next foods can certainly help in the detoxification process.

1. Fruits & vegetables

Due to the high levels of fiber, fruits and vegetables will digest quickly. Additionally, people withdrawing or detoxing from alcoholic beverages may often crave sweets. Fruits contain glucose, which can match the craving for something nice without weighing too greatly on the person's belly since appetite will decrease through the cleansing stage. Relating to Mayoclinic.com, some fruits and vegetables include raspberries, pears, oranges, strawberries, bananas, and figs.

2. Whole grains

Carbohydrates are essential for recovery, as they offer dietary fiber and energy that your detoxer may be lacking. Processed grains such as white bread also provide carbohydrates for energy but are a less healthy option in the long-run. Wholegrain contains more dietary fiber, leading to feeling fuller rather than causing your body any digestive issues.

3. Anything containing vitamin B

Continuous alcohol consumption leads to too little vitamin B. vitamin B is vital in the body to replenish the body's supply. Foods saturated in vitamin B include salmon, broccoli, asparagus, and romaine lettuce.

4. Proteins lower in fat

Many alcoholics in detoxification will have a reduced appetite or just be switched off by food, but foods saturated in fiber can help them feel full. Protein with zero fat content is ideal because they favorably affect feeling and energy, resulting in less potential for relapse. Such foods include seafood and lean meat.

5. Cayenne pepper

Though it might not sound appealing, adding cayenne pepper to foods can reduce alcohol cravings and increase appetite. That is beneficial because in detoxification, the desire tends to be suppressed, and essential nutrients aren't received. Cayenne pepper can also assist in decreasing alcohol drawback symptoms such as nausea.

Though making sure to eat these food types during detox won't ensure hanging around, they'll likely ease the discomfort and urges that accompany the detox stage.

Foods To Avoid During Detox

Sugars

Extreme sugar consumption causes prolonged cravings, lethargy, anxiety, and chemical substance imbalances. Also, it often creates a new kind of addiction for individuals in recovery.

Caffeine

It overstimulates the central nervous system, which can result in stress and insomnia, both of which may be detrimental to effective cleansing and recovery.

Prepared or artificial foods such as rubbish or junk food

For this reason, the liver must work much harder to breakdown preservatives and chemicals within these kinds of foods, and also you want to permit the liver to rest whenever you can during detoxification and early recovery.

Chapter 7

5 Methods for Detoxing from Alcohol

Alcoholism is a significant disease that should receive medical assistance. Yet, only around 10 to 20 percent of individuals experiencing alcohol drawback receive treatment based on the American Academy of Family Doctors.

Whatever the known reasons why people don't undergo treatment, it is imperative to sobriety. So, when you are lamenting over lost associations, money, or careers credited to alcoholism, or even though you think that perhaps you drink too much, cleansing might be considered an excellent option for you. Below are a few tips to get clean and sober and complete alcoholic beverages detoxification successfully.

1) Make an idea and commit to quit

An essential component in getting sober and going right through detox is to produce an arrangement for sobriety. While people can reap the benefits of involuntary cleansing and treatment, your recovery will primarily rely on your determination to improve.

In such, you should be ready to make a changeover from your present life to detoxification, and then transition again into culture. Call us at Alta Mira Recovery to find out more about alcoholic beverages detoxing and what treatment options are used, as well as how long you'll be likely to maintain detox. Some cleansing programs last a couple of days, while some can take up to a week or even more. Facilities often use medications to aid severe addiction instances, so know about your options.

2) Understand the withdrawal symptoms.

Going right through detoxification doesn't mean you won't experience withdrawal symptoms, mainly if you are a long-term or substantial consumer of alcohol. The Improvements in Psychiatric Treatment journal cites that patients ought to know what things to expect during the drawback, and exactly how those symptoms can be treated. Knowledge is the main element here. Common alcoholic beverages drawback medical indications include:

- Depression

- Anxiety

- Irritability or restlessness

- Exhaustion or insomnia

- Seizures or delirium tremens (DTs)

- Urges for alcohol

- Sweating

- Physical weakness

3) Understand that detox is an initial step.

Some believe that cleansing is one procedure, and one is fine to re-integrate into society and stop taking in once and for all; this isn't quite so. Detoxification is only a preliminary part of the healing process. An extensive treatment solution will ensure that detoxification is utilized in tandem with other treatment methods like cognitive behavioral therapy.

4) Find new meaning in your life.

A deterrent to the people seeking help for alcoholic beverages is that they think their life might not be as enjoyable without it. Experience can be fun, enjoyable, and utterly advantageous without alcoholic beverages! Explore different therapies like artwork, music, yoga exercise, or trekking to find new, healthy ways to take pleasure from life. Besides, it could be fun when you awaken with a killer hangover, and you also can't keep in mind what you did last night?

5) Change your daily diet and workout program.

The use of alcoholic beverages and the next withdrawal period can result in a person to be dehydrated, so drink a lot of water. Additionally, alcoholic beverages can deplete your body of essential nutrition and damage vital organs. Get the body right again by nourishing it with foods abundant with minerals and vitamins and by working out. Proper maintenance of the body leaves you refreshed as well as your brain clear (healthy bodywork). To make an idea to quit alcoholic beverages, make an idea to nurture the body as well.

Considering alcoholic beverages, detox is a superb first rung on the ladder in a lifelong intent to get sober. Alta Mira Recovery is certified to treat alcoholic beverages withdrawal symptoms and offer continuous care. Give us a call today to find out more about our service and how we will exactly help you get over alcoholism or alcoholic beverages abuse. Your daily life won't be lost without alcoholic drinks. Your brand-new life can start once you forget about your dependence.

www.ingramcontent.com/pod-product-compliance
Lightning Source LLC
Chambersburg PA
CBHW071117030426
42336CB00013BA/2129